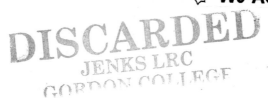
Gone Without A Trace

BY

MARIANNE DICKERMAN CALDWELL

Elder Books
Forest Knolls, California

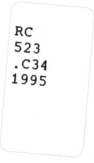
Library of Congress Cataloging in Publication Data

Main Entry Under Title:
Gone Without A Trace
Caldwell, Marianne

1. Alzheimer's disease 2. Aged 3. Loss 4. Adoption
5. Missing persons

LCCN 94-061037
ISBN 0-943873-24-X

Printed in the United States of America
Cover Photograph: Marianne Caldwell
Cover Design: Bonnie Fisk-Hayden

CONTENTS

TO NANCY

WHOSE
COMPASSION AND WISDOM
HAS BEEN AN INSPIRATION TO ME

ACKNOWLEDGMENTS

Gone Without A Trace grew from the anguish and despair which engulfed my spirit in the years following my mother's disappearance. It has been a journey which I could not have done alone. My deepest appreciation goes to Nancy Verrier, my psychotherapist, who has been a constant source of encouragement and inspiration. It is because of her that I have dared to face my grief, raw as it was.

For the past two years, I have received great comfort and support from my brothers William and Bob, who have known, too, the despairing experience of our mother vanishing. Over the years I have been so glad that it is them, I call and know, as brothers. I acknowledge my uncle, Robert W. Mallory and family for their love and understanding.

I especially want to thank Eileen E. Rogers, Janet Herman-Bertsch, Dennie Caldwell, Kathy Stern, Don Gentner, Dr. Judith Stewart, Margaret Wentworth Owings, Joycelyn King, and my young friend, Mara Boyd. All have been exceptional in their friendship to me throughout this time; all have cheered me on **to write my story.**

My thanks to the following professionals who have been supportive and generous with their time: Dr. Jeff Durbin, Maryanne Wilson, and Sandy Fortier. Corporal Bruce Mathews of the New Hampshire State Police Headquarters has always responded with professionalism and kindness. I am also grateful to Lieutenant Gerald Bernier of the N.H. Fish & Game Department for organizing the initial search mission.

And finally, as a loving tribute to my mother, remembering how much she gave of herself to others, and to me, **Gone Without A Trace** is written. None of us know today what happened the day she disappeared. All who knew her hope the ending was benevolent and peaceful, and of the sort she might have wished for herself. This surely is what she deserved, and what we would all have wished for her.

INTRODUCTION

Most people believe that having a family member vanish
will never happen to them. Those who fall victim to this
trauma consequently are caught unaware about what to
do. No one is exempt from the possibility of it happening
to them. Each year in the United States, approximately
1.8 million persons are reported missing. Many remain
missing. My mother is one of them.

Ironically, it was on Friday the13th that my adoptive
mother, Stella Mallory Dickerman, an Alzheimer's disease victim, vanished. I never imagined that this would
be the first day of more than a thousand to come without
knowing what happened to her. In the years since her
disappearance, I have experienced firsthand the feelings
of profound grief, anguish and confusion that engulf one
when faced with the **unknown.**

Although literature is available on how to find persons
who willfully disappear, there is little information on
what to do when you need to mobilize a search for a

memory-impaired adult. Families are at the mercy of others when dealing with grave crises such as an abducted child or a cognitively impaired adult who mysteriously vanishes. This book provides guidelines for contacting appropriate agencies when someone vanishes, and it offers examples of inquiries to be circulated for locating a missing person. It also describes the pitfalls that can occur while dealing with law enforcement agencies when someone vanishes.

Gone Without A Trace describes the trauma of having a loved one disappear: the profundity of grief when there can be no closure, as well as the connection felt with others who have lost loved ones through tragic and sometimes mysterious circumstances. This story is written in the hope that it may help others understand and face some of the unexpected and torturous losses which may come their way as they journey through life.

PORTRAIT OF
STELLA MALLORY DICKERMAN

During the nineteen twenties when few Americans and
very few women attended college, Stella Mallory earned
a bachelor's degree at Oberlin College in Ohio and
moved to Michigan to become an art teacher. Like most
American women in the thirties, she became a wife and
mother, devoting her time to making a home for her
family.

In the course of the forties, after giving birth to a second
son and taking a young daughter into her home, Stella
became through separation and divorce, a single parent
with three small children. While employed as a teacher,
she returned to college to earn her master's degree, and
through the adoption of her daughter, became one of the
first single parents to adopt a child.

During the fifties, she became an instructor in art educa-
tion at a major university and later the art supervisor for

a large public school system, all the while providing a stable and comfortable home for her three children. When her children completed school in the sixties and went off on their own, Stella continued her career as a public school administrator. In addition, she devoted numerous volunteer hours to her church and community and explored her abilities as an artist.

In the later part of the seventies and eighties, Stella retired from her career and became involved in international programs, helping refugees settle in the United States. She travelled extensively to record in water colors the cultures and landscapes of Europe, Asia, and North America.

As the nineties approached, Stella's cognitive abilities began to decline. Although physically healthy, she began showing signs of forgetfulness, such as leaving ingredients out of recipes when she baked. Her paintings began to look primitive. On occasion, she confused her son with her brother and did not remember she had a daughter. It was during this time that she began to forget where she was walking if she set out to do something. She was diagnosed as having dementia, probably Alzheimer's Disease.

On Friday, September the 13th, 1991, at the age of eighty three, Stella went for a walk. How far she walked or what she was thinking is unknown, because she was never seen again.

Stella Dickerman lived a long, full life and did it all at a time when most women were limited to very narrow roles. She was a traditional wife and she was a single parent. She was a mother who cooked and baked from scratch and ate three meals a day with her children. She was a successful and respected career woman at a time when administrative positions were almost always given to men. She was an artist who mastered the complexities of water colors at a time when most painters settled for oils. And she was a generous, caring, and much loved friend to her family and the many people who had the good fortune to know her as neighbor, fellow-worker, and teacher.

How could a woman with so many abilities and personal strengths decline so drastically in her last few years? Cruelly, that is what happens to those who get Alzheimer's disease. But how could she disappear so suddenly and completely? **That is what no one knows.**

Horror Of The News: My Story

To have a Mother vanish without a trace
is an unnerving experience.
One which I long for to end.

On Friday, September 13, 1991, Stella Dickerman disappeared from a children's boarding school near Rindge, New Hampshire. For my older brother Bob, my younger brother William and me, our mother, a friend, teacher, artist, and Alzheimer's victim had vanished. The following words were spoken by William at the remembrance service four months following her disappearance:

We can celebrate her life, and yet, the ending still makes us all very sad. It was a sunny afternoon. She was surrounded by school children whom she liked to watch. There were carpenters working both inside and outside of the house, yet they didn't see her, although somehow she seems to have circled the house *and gotten back to the dirt road. **Then nothing more.** Probably that night she perished. And those few hours before that are the ones that cause us the most grief and sadness. She must have been hopelessly lost, long before it got dark and cold. Those hours must have been filled with fear, loneliness, and confusion as she wondered why no one came to help her.*

The mysterious disappearance of my mother in a densely forested region of New Hampshire has left many questions unanswered. I am beginning to understand the impact of having a mother disappear. Not once but twice, as I am an adoptee.

It is the more recent trauma which has erupted in me all the feelings associated with my original wrenching separation from my birth mother. The feelings of helplessness, confusion, grief, and shame which spewed at the time of my mother's vanishing are the same feelings I experienced as an infant when I was abandoned. Both losses have been devastating events over which I had no control, and as a result, both have left my spirit aching.

Early Saturday morning on September 14, 1991, I was awakened by a phonecall from my brother William. I was chilled by his words, "Mother is lost!" He went on to say that she had walked away from the children's softball game the previous evening and hadn't been seen since.

Although stunned, I managed to remain calm while William told me that police with bloodhounds were in the woods looking for her all night. The search would continue throughout the forested region today and later a helicopter would fly overhead, scanning below the thousands of forested acres surrounding the country school.

When I hung up, I realized that the unimaginable had happened to me. In one single moment of time, my world darkened and I was again thrust by a thunderous force into a despairing and haunting experience. I felt overcome by a sense of surrealness and fear.

I promptly arranged to take emergency leave from my work as a Nurse to join my brothers in the search. I work with military veterans hospitalized for psychiatric treatment of Post-Traumatic Stress Disorder. Although I deal with patients suffering from traumatic events, I was completely unprepared for what would happen to me. Suddenly in shock from my own personal trauma, I felt utterly overwhelmed.

3

Searching For Answers

Within a few hours, I left San Francisco on a flight bound for Boston, clutching a few recent photos of my mother in my hand. I arrived at the airport at midnight and was met by a friend. Throughout the night, we stopped at every hospital along the sixty mile route from Boston to Rindge, New Hampshire.

Nervously, I presented the photos at each Emergency Room, asking if anyone fitting my mother's description was brought in for treatment. Feelings of consternation mounted within me as nurses in one hospital after another shook their heads and responded, "No one like your mother has been brought in tonight."

Shortly after daylight, we arrived at the boarding school. As we turned onto the dirt lane leading to the school, tree after tree was marked by a blue ribbon, indicating that a search team had passed this way. At the softball field where my mother was last seen, the search and rescue command center buzzed with activity.

My older brother Bob was engrossed in the search activity while William fielded questions from television and newspaper reporters. We spoke only briefly. The urgency of the search and rescue mission hampered us from acknowledging our emotions.

Multiple volunteers, search dogs, police, emergency medical teams, and fire fighters were present, all involved in the massive search. Paramedics emerged from an Army helicopter, carrying an empty gurney. Tears filled my eyes. All day, the helicopter with its distinct sound made back and forth sweeps over the densely wooded forest.

Although stunned, I recall speaking to one individual after another, thanking them for being there and participating in the ground search. All the while my eyes strained as I scanned the surrounding woods, desperately searching for a clue.

Looking back, I realize that I wasn't really interacting with all that was going on; I was numb, struggling to organize my thoughts and make sense of events around me.

Soon, temperatures reached ninety sunny degrees, in contrast to the night Mother disappeared when heavy rains fell, fierce winds blew, and the temperature was in the low forties. People returned to the command site exhausted and drenched in perspiration from trudging through marsh, blackberry brush, dense foliage, and thick branches in the intense heat. Vans were marked as rescue units and more bloodhounds and air-sniff dogs wearing orange vests arrived.

When sunset came, the search ended and the dogs took over. It was crushing to watch the evening television report showing a photo of our mother surrounded by her watercolor paintings and hear about the grim wilderness search on her behalf.

Gripping events unfolded over the following days. A police detective arrived with the news that there were several sightings of my mother. One woman claimed to have seen her as she was nearing Route 119, one mile from the school. Another man came forth saying she had flagged him down in his truck on the lane adjacent to the school. He recalled her saying, "I have been trying all day to find the white house." He pointed down the dirt lane in the direction of one of the school buildings where there is a white house. She replied, "Thank you, thank you... you are my savior, just like my son." He described Mother as looking fatigued and unsteady. Another man claimed to have seen and spoken to her on the highway, but he refused to give his name.

Police informed us that they released an all-points bulletin (APB) and entered her name into the National Crime

Information Center for Missing Persons. Sadly, many months later, I learned that the bulletin was apparently never released, and instead, an "attempt to locate" radio bulletin was issued.

Over the following days, more television coverage was aired in Ohio, near her former residence of Oberlin, from where she had moved two weeks before her disappearance. I drove around New Hampshire, Massachusetts and Vermont distributing flyers and making inquiries at hospitals, shelters, police stations, senior centers and other social service agencies.

It was uncanny to pass newsstands and see headlines: *Alzheimer's Victim Missing Since Friday; Authorities Baffled, RINDGE Woman Still Missing; Elderly Woman Vanishes: Anything Could Have Happened; A Private Eye Is Looking for Missing Woman; Woman's Disappearance Remains A Mystery.* It was jarring to see her photo posted everywhere: on business windows, doors, posts, and trees. Each time I drove, the radio announced the latest news from the search. Constantly I asked myself: **How could this have happened?**

Mistaken Identity

A week after the search began, I returned to California, having been awake for well over twenty four hours. I felt immense heavy-heartedness from the week's events and the unsuccessful search, now in the seventh day.

The flight home was a misadventure. Because my return ticket was standby, I anticipated some delay at the airport, but nothing like what I encountered. After waiting several hours I was boarded on a direct flight to the West Coast. Shortly after, the plane was directed back to the boarding gate and the flight was cancelled due to a mechanical difficulty. For the next several hours, we remained within the departure gate. Finally, it was announced that those of us with standby tickets would be unable to depart until the following day.

Despite being nearly exhausted, I was unable to nap. My thoughts were fixated on the search efforts and my mother's whereabouts. Throughout the night, I made phone inquiries to hospitals and shelters listed in the Yellow Pages. The following day I finally boarded a flight for San Francisco.

While awaiting take off, I sorrowfully reflected how the plane would be flying over the search area. I felt disheartened and anxious at the thought of flying westward, away from the dreary search site.

Several hours later, upon arriving in Las Vegas, I had a terrifying emotional experience. I suddenly saw a woman whom I thought was my mother being assisted by a flight attendant to an area marked "Security". The woman was elderly, small in stature, wearing a blue nylon jacket like my mother wore at the time she disappeared, and holding a cane which resembled my mother's walking stick. She looked my way, and then was quickly out of sight, having passed through the Security door.

I became frantic and desperate to reach her. Immediately I approached an attendant, crying and pleading to let me go through. I pulled out an article describing the search now in progress. I felt totally confused, knowing I was in Las Vegas and the improbability of my mother being in the airport. Yet remembering how she loved to travel, I was believing for the moment that the stranger was my mother.

The airline personnel responded to me in a way which

was remarkably understanding. A telephone call was placed to the administrative offices. Soon afterwards, the elderly woman, accompanied by a flight attendant, was brought back to where I was standing. The small woman who now stood before me smiled and said nothing.

Immediately, when face to face with her, I realized she was not my mother. I sat down in a nearby seat and wept, all the while clutching the newspaper article in my hand. I realized then how desperately I yearned for my mother to be found.

ALONE

Mother's disappearance is by far the most gruelling emotional experience of my adult life. The lack of resolution pervades my thoughts and I have barely slept since she disappeared. Each night I go over and over the same disturbing questions: If someone picked her up, why? And why haven't they come forth? If foul play, what could be the motive?

People rarely mention what has happened and act as if I should be feeling better. Although some co-workers are empathetic, others have voiced annoyance with me for being unable to go one with my life. Some have said nothing at all.

Occasionally, people make strange comments such as: "Now you can begin to have closure," or "I imagine she died peacefully in the woods." I keep saying it is not natural to have a parent lost, missing in the woods. She may be alive somewhere, not dead.

I feel frustrated and misunderstood when people say: "I know just how you feel. I have suffered loss, too. I am divorced," or, "I know what it is to lose a parent; my mother died, too." I want to scream, "You don't know what I am feeling! You may have experienced the death of a loved one, but you had a body to grieve over and know the circumstances of the death." I used to feel a part of the work team. Now I've lost that connection, too.

I miss being geographically close to my mid-western friends, having relocated to the west coast only two years ago. These friends, with whom I have shared decades of history, knew Mother as a person in wellness, and finally as an Alzheimer's victim.

My brother and I talk daily. Today he spoke about finding it helpful to be close to the search activity and available for police reports. Hundreds of letters, cards, and phone calls have been received from friends and well-wishers. Sometimes I wonder if I am imagining all that has happened. The situation might seem less surreal if I could be close to the search activity.

The latest report from the search site is that members of a search dog team are at the school, studying reports and charting a course for another ground search. I am holding onto the hope she will be found. Then the next major crisis will begin: what condition will she be in when they find her?

It is painful to go to work during this time. I have the feeling of a compressing band around my head many times each day. Every time the phone rings, I am hoping the call is for me, as I anxiously wait for answers. I'm afraid that if I disclose my feelings, I'll be deemed weak, not in control. I don't know how one comes to grips with this kind of trauma or if I'm strong enough to deal with the experience. I seek out supportive friends whenever I feel flooded with grief.

I have a surge of hope again. My brother phoned to say that searchers brought in a dog team again to the area of Stump Pond on school grounds. The dog barked in a way which indicated there might be a lead. Television reporters were on site, filming the fireman diver who was following the lead. The fireman dived the south end of the pond, but found nothing. God, I feel pumped up with hope again.

I have yet to meet anyone who has ever been through the experience of having someone vanish and remain unfound. Sometimes the pain of having had two mothers disappear feels almost more than I can bear. I constantly wonder whether she is alive in a shelter or a hospital, remaining unidentified. My deepest fear is that she will not be found and I will be consumed by the unknown.

On the Eve of returning to the search center in New Hampshire for the second time, I made the following journal entry:

Dear Mother:

I am preparing a tiny box of treasures to take to New Hampshire for you, to bury it where you were last reported seen. The days since your disappearance seem unreal. My heart and soul anguish to find you. I go over and over where you might be and what could have happened. I wonder if I will get through this stressful time—quite frankly, if I'll survive.

In my lifetime I never imagined I would be looking for you so intensely. Now the hope of finding you is diminishing with each passing week. I never wanted you to be afraid in life. I only wanted you to be safe in your illness and to pass out of this life quietly and gently. I hope we will soon know where you are. I love you... I miss you... I want to find you...

Your daughter, Marianne

31

GONE WITHOUT A TRACE

The search is now in its fifty-third day and I feel relieved to be back at the search site. My brother and I walked miles today along the dirt lane and trails in search of a clue. We came across a single plastic bag with a rock inside. Knowing that our mother liked stones and that she sometimes carried a plastic bag in her pocket, we carefully brought our find home. Thinking this might be a clue, we combed the surrounding area, but nothing more was found.

Yesterday, authorities brought in a plane and Air National Guard troops for a final big search effort. Search and rescue ground teams retraced areas searched weeks ago. Divers with underwater cameras from New York State explored the deepest part of the lower pond while the upper pond was drained as they searched for evidence. With the black German canine on alert, private detectives canoed and probed the edges of the lower pond.

Snow is predicted to fall next week. Hunting season begins on Wednesday. Signs are posted on trees around the school warning: "No hunting allowed; No trespassing." It seems doubtful that a hunter will come across her remains.

Mother's plight has taken a different turn. The possibility of foul play is increasing greatly. All this is so perplexing. I can't stand the thought of foul play. I feel like kicking the wall...my car...anything. Where is she? I feel scared, sad, and angry and unnerved by my vulnerability.

It has been more than two years now since the day my mother disappeared. I continue to ponder the question, "What could have happened?" Although the initial search went on almost continuously for several months, volunteer efforts continued on an informal basis for much longer. Somehow, in a matter of a few minutes she completely disappeared, leaving no trace.

While my journey out of total despair has been a long one, filled with pain and complicated by the unknowns, I am confident that someday I will be able to make sense of what still seems so utterly senseless.

I feel humbled by the extraordinary efforts of the many persons who unselfishly participated in the immediate search. Of all who helped, only the small Country School community knew our mother personally, for she moved there from Ohio only two weeks before she vanished. A few of them had known her before Alzheimer's disease had taken its toll on her talents and strengths. The others who came and assisted in the search knew only that a fellow human being was lost and that help was needed. My mother had helped many when she could. Now others were generous when she was in need.

Unresolved Grief:

When a Person Remains Missing

If we do recognize that someone has suffered a loss, one that we cannot ignore such as the death of a parent, spouse, or child, we can only tolerate the bereaved person's grief for so long and then we expect him or her to "get on with life". Grieving people need to be given the permission to feel their loss and the time to process it. These are people who are suffering as a result of society's ignorance, and its use of denial as a major defense against pain and paradox.

Nancy Verrier

The first four months following my mother's disappearance were spent assiduously making contacts to everywhere I imagined might bring answers. When search endeavors failed, my brother and I began to make plans for a Remembrance Service, hoping this would bring closure and a sense of peace and allow us to go on with our lives. Wrong! Instead, I became haunted in various ways by the unknown. My spirit fluctuated between agonizing despair and fear that the unknown would last forever. I felt totally helpless.

What I didn't understand was that my reaction was **normal** to an **abnormal** event. Nancy Verrier, a leading expert in the field of adoption, sums it up as follows: "If the primal experience for the adopted child is abandonment, then the core issues are loss and the fear of a further abandonment."

To be grief stricken leaves one feeling raw and vulnerable. It is imperative to realize that these feelings are valid. Grieving is a time when one feels completely detached from persons and events around them. As the focus shifts inwards, one becomes desensitized to external events or persons outside oneself.

When a loved one remains missing, the bereaved will be in a state of perpetual grief. It is impossible to bring closure without knowledge of what happened and without the presence of a body. How can one conceptualize what it is they are grieving when there are no answers? Raphael has described the situation as follows: "Since so many of the losses are invisible or unrecognized, the customary rituals of mourning provide little consolation." (Herman, 1992).

Many persons in Western society are uncomfortable when faced with a person who is grieving and in mourning after the death of a loved one. Is it any wonder then, that when there is no body, grief becomes complicated, unresolved, and often misunderstood?

People often cannot bear to witness the anguish of people who are dealing with traumatic loss. "Outsiders" to intense grief cannot know the depth of trauma experienced by "insiders". This shared understanding explains the intense feelings of connection with other people in a like situation.

The process of healing is slow and seems to be marked universally by a sense that one is alone in grief and deadened to feeling anything relating to another person. The case is similar with suicide. According to Lukas and Seiden (1987), "Suicide survivors suffer because: they are grieving for a dead person, because they are suffering from a traumatic experience, because people don't talk about suicide, and the silence that surrounds it gets in the way of the healing that comes with normal mourning."

Silence also prevails when someone remains missing. People don't know what to say in these circumstances and often say nothing. Co-workers and friends should try to acknowledge the loss in whatever way they can. When this doesn't happen, survivors feel hurt, resentful, and disconnected to those around them and the sense of aloneness is intensified.

Sometimes people avoid the subject of the missing person because they fear that talking about it will trigger more grieving. What is most misunderstood is that the thought of the person missing is always on one's mind. The anxious anticipation of news of the loved one is constant.

People in a perpetual state of grief experience intrusive images and memories associated with the time when the person vanished. They experience spontaneous and unwanted recall of the event, suddenly acting or feeling as if it were reoccurring.

I found myself triggered by the environment over and over. On days when it rained, I would spontaneously visualize my mother out in the woods, wet and cold. Whenever I drove past a forested region, I would scan it, looking for a clue. Looking deep into the forested area in search of clothing or objects, I would imagine the searchers in New Hampshire doing the same. Whenever a police care or ambulance passed, my heart would skip a beat, and once again, the same feelings of fear, and hopelessness that I had experienced during the long search and rescue efforts would resurface.

I was inundated by intrusive thoughts: was she dead in the woods, had she been given a ride out of the area and let out, and finally, was she a victim of foul play? All of these thoughts were haunting. I spoke only to a select few friends about my wrenching emotional pain. I couldn't envision anything worse than living with the unknown, to lose a mother, now, for a second time.

I have come to believe that it doesn't matter what the trauma is. All survivors of victims, whether they be related to homicide, suicide, MIA (Missing In Action), or those who have been orphaned, ask "Why?" Survivors, then, become victims themselves. Their feeling of being victimized is universal when struggling to make sense of something so out of the ordinary. One thing is known for certain: no person is immune to the unimaginable happening to them, and I suspect that no one can prepare for such a trauma.

Following the first anniversary of my mother's disappearance, I found a psychotherapist whose expertise is working with individuals who have suffered devastating losses. Finding a therapist who truly understands the profundity of grief when someone vanishes is in itself a challenge. I knew firsthand, as a result of my encounters with others, how difficult it is for someone to have an understanding of complicated bereavement issues unless they have experienced it or have been educated about it.

Simple bereavement is defined as a reaction to loss, followed by feelings of depression, loss of appetite, weight loss and insomnia. Additional guilt, if present, is usually about things done or not done at the time of death. In the literature, there is little written about how complicated bereavement manifests for individuals dealing with the disappearance of a loved one. As a result of my own experience and in talking with others who have been faced with a similar tragedy, I recognize how profound bereavement is under these circum-stances. The suddenness of a person vanishing, and not knowing what has happened disallows the **finality** of death. It is all the customary feelings associated with simple bereavement and it is **without an ending.**

One speculates continuously, "If I just make the right call to the right person, I'll solve this mystery. If I just look in the right place, I'll find the person". And "If I stop look-ing, the person may never be found". These are the lingering and troubling thoughts of people dealing with the **unknown**, which is the core of complicated bereavement when someone remains missing.

Many people have assumptions about the grieving process and how long it should take. There are often up-spoken expectations that the individual should recover from irrevocable loss within a relatively brief period of time. If grieving people fail to meet this assigned time frame, they are often regarded in a negative way. John Bowlby has described the situation as follows:

Loss of a loved person is one of the most intensely painful experiences any human being can suffer. And not only is it painful to experience but it is also painful to witness, if only because we are so impotent to help. To the bereaved, nothing but the return of the lost person can bring true comfort; if what we provide falls short of that, it is felt almost as an insult. There is a tendency to underestimate how intensely distressing and disabling loss usually is and for how long the distress, and often the disablement, commonly lasts. Conversely, there is a tendency to suppose that a healthy person can and should get over a bereavement not only fairly rapidly but also completely.

In our Western culture, it is common to admire people who appear to be dealing well with grief for their strength of character. They are often commended for carrying on with their usual activities. The truth is that responding as if no loss or trauma occurred more likely indicates denial or an avoidance of dealing with the trauma.

People are often unaware of the changes in the grieving person's perception of the world when there is no body. For many in traumatic grief, the world is no longer a safe place to be. They know that someone can disappear and that terrifying things can happen. According to Judith Herman (1992), "Traumatic events are extraordinary not because they occur rarely, but rather because they overwhelm the ordinary human adaptation to life." Although I had suffered a trauma, I didn't know the degree to which the suddenness of my mother vanishing and remaining unfound would empty me of my coping strengths and how profound my sense of helplessness would be. I struggled to ask for what I needed. After all, **what I felt I needed** was only for my mother to be found.

It wasn't until one year later that I had my first conversations with others who have a loved one missing and presumed dead. Most spoke about feeling that they were frozen in time, frozen at the traumatic moment when their loved one vanished. Some mirrored my own sentiment that the most difficult aspect of coping is the feeling that no one can understand how gripping and heart wrenching the pain is.

For families who have a child or adult member missing under mysterious circumstances, the suffering is beyond what any human being should have to endure. The greatest gift we can give them is to try to understand how unnerving it must be to live with the unknown. The way to do this is through **LOVE**. In other words:

LISTEN: Listen to what the person is saying—he or she is entitled to their feelings. Remember that feelings are generated from one's life experiences and may differ from yours. That's okay.

OBSERVE: What does the person want to say, but is afraid to put out, for example, his or her worst fears?

VALIDATE: Let the person know that what they are feeling is normal. It is the traumatic experience which is abnormal.

EMPATHIZE: Offer compassion and sensitivity.

Healing takes time and becomes a personal journey for each person courageous enough to truly face their grief. As Viktor E. Frankl wrote in **Man's Search For Meaning:** *He who has a why to live can bear with almost any how.*

8

WHEN
A COGNITIVELY IMPAIRED
PERSON BECOMES LOST

I fidget and I fuss
I go in circles hunting something
I pass right by it!
I get tight—I get frantic.
Calm down, calm down.
Get your self outdoors,
Make up a destination.
Look around you.
Smile at the folks along the way.
Whee, I'm feeling better!
I take a deep breath—
Look skyward and say,
Thank you, God!

Stella M. Dickerman (1990)

To most of us, memory loss is something we relate to with annoyance or, at best, with humor. How often does someone misplace something or forget a prearranged meeting and humorously say, "Oh, I must be getting Alzheimer's." To those effected by Alzheimer's disease, memory loss is anything but humorous.

According to statistics compiled by the Alzheimer's Association, four million Americans have lost their capacity to recognize familiar places and faces. Many become unable to remember their names and eventually lose their ability to speak meaningfully. Although their cognition is impaired, their physical condition typically remains unaffected for years. They can't remember or make decisions, but they can walk, often vigorously.

Alzheimer's patients have a propensity to become confused and to wander. What actually causes these patients to wander is unknown. However, it is theorized that wandering may be a result of disorientation or restlessness. This unpredictable behavior can result in a dangerous situation for memory-impaired people when they travel or use public transportation. Caregivers are challenged to find ways in which they can allow the patients' freedom to move about, yet maintain an environment which is safe for them.

An Alzheimer's patient may feel lost much of the time when out of his or her familiar environment and wandering may be an expression of finding the way home to recover control. Many get lost in local shopping malls and even in the neighborhoods in which they live. The Alzheimer's patient on the move can be regarded as simply searching for something familiar, but must be recognized as vulnerable.

The first forty-eight hours are the most critical for persons who are lost, for it is during this time that chances for their being returned alive are greatest. And it is during these same hours when their families' feelings of hope are greatest for their safe return. During these hours family members are in urgent need of support and assistance. Family, friends, and volunteers need to expeditiously mobilize and participate in search efforts for the lost person. It is important to keep a telephone line open so that the primary parties can be notified in the event that the missing person has been found.

It was not until 1993, eighteen months after my mother's disappearance, that the ALZHEIMER SAFE RETURN program was developed. This is a nationwide program designed to locate and return to safety missing persons with Alzheimer's disease. Families register their memory-impaired relative with this program and the patient receives an identification bracelet, wallet card, and clothing labels. Their names are entered into a national database. This enables police, community agencies and private citizens to identify people with Alzheimer's disease and helps return them home.

The Alzheimer's Association is increasing its efforts to educate the public about the wandering behavior of people with Alzheimer's disease and the services available nationwide through the Safe Return program. Fortunately, most crises related to a demented individual becoming lost are quickly resolved. Demented persons who become lost and stressed often lose the ability to remember their own name, address, or telephone number. They may be completely unable to ask for assistance. An identification bracelet is of great help in this situation. A recent photo of the individual should be readily accessible.

If the police show resistance to assist in the search, the caregiver must alert them as to how grave it is for a demented individual to be lost. Caregivers have sometimes been told that a Missing Person Report cannot be filed until twenty four hours after the disappearance. **This information is false.** It is imperative to contact authorities immediately and to verify that the information entered into police records is accurate and complete.

My own experience alerts me to the difficulties in working with small police departments. It is often difficult to obtain verification of information entered into police reports. The smaller police agencies in villages and rural towns may be restricted by limited financial resources. Training for officers may be minimal and their knowledge of what to do when an individual vanishes is frequently limited. Often they are unable to respond effectively and this is deeply frustrating for families. Concerns should be expressed immediately if problems arise.

Once a cognitively impaired person has been gone more than twenty-four hours, publicity is crucial. Local television stations and newspapers are usually eager to alert the public to the plight of the missing person. Flyers displaying a recent photo help generate public concern. Surrounding hospitals should be contacted as well as nursing homes, shelters, mental health facilities, law enforcement agencies, or any other place a rescuer may bring a confused stranger.

It is essential to prepare a written profile of the lost person as soon after the disappearance as possible. This should list the time and whereabouts of the disappearance, as well as the person's behavior, mannerisms, and conversation topics. Appendices 2 and 3 highlight the precise information needed in a search profile.

Most lost persons are found. For many however, the disappearance marks the beginning of a long and grim search which may span days, weeks, months, and years before answers come. Sometimes, answers may never

come. Family members must follow their intuitive feelings about what they believe might have happened and
check out the possibilities.

Finding Informaton
About Unidentified Persons

"Within the United States annually an estimated 1.8 million persons are reported missing."
Ted Gunderson

In his book, **How To Locate Anyone Anywhere**, Ted Gunderson professes that the majority of persons disappearing have done so willfully. He calculates that persons in the United States disappear because they:

(1) clearly want to be wherever they are;

(2) have no home, literally or figuratively;

(3) are being held somehow against their will;

(4) are victims of homicide, suicide, accident, or unattended, maybe unrecorded, natural death.

Families who suspect that the person's disappearance is due to memory impairment or some other unexplained cause such as death, abduction, or foul play, may find police departments impersonal. Budget restraints and overwork are commonly used explanations for the laissez-faire attitude which often prevails within police departments. To distraught families, such excuses are inimical to peace of mind when someone remains missing. My advice is to be persistent and ask for what you need, even if you must do so, again and again.

The Federal Bureau of Investigation (FBI) maintains the National Crime Information Center (NCIC) system with headquarters in Washington D.C. This computerized system holds, among other data, the names of missing persons and their personal descriptors. The NCIC system is available to most law enforcement agencies nationally. A request by a non-relative or family member to enter the name of a missing person cannot be denied. **It is the law!** If any law enforcement agency refuses your request, contact the nearest FBI office for assistance.

All missing and unidentified persons should be listed in the NCIC computer. Once recorded, law enforcement agencies throughout the country have access to the missing person's personal identifiers, including his or her age, medical condition, and dental information. In the event a law enforcement agency were to find an individual who did not know his or her name, the agency could enter personal identifiers to accurately identify the individual. All persons entered into the NCIC computer are automatically cross-referenced in an effort to match up persons known to be missing with unidentified found persons or bodies.

Once an originating agency has entered the name of a missing person into the NCIC computer, the agency is then responsible for entering the Missing Person Data Collection File. This file details information obtained from the missing person's doctor, dentist, and family. The file includes the following information:

[1] *Initial report which is completed by the reporting officer and entered into the NCIC.*

[2] *List of Personal Descriptors: to be completed by parent/ legal guardian/next of kin and returned to the originating agency.*

[3] *Medical Forms: (name of missing person, date of birth, and authorization to release records on medical information, optic and dental history information forms). The forms must be completed by the missing person's physician, dentist, and optician and returned by a parent, legal guardian, or next of kin to the police agency which completed the original report. Caregivers should return the completed forms to the reporting officer. The information is then added to the missing person's*

record on file in the NCIC computer.

Criteria for entry into the Missing Person file:

(1)   Disability-A person of any age who is missing and under proven physical/mental disability or is senile (sic), thereby subjecting himself/herself or others to personal and immediate danger.

(2)   Endangered - A person of any age who is missing and in the company of another person under circumstances indicating that his/her physical safety is in danger.

(3)   Involuntary - A person of any age who is missing under circumstances indicating that the disappearance was not voluntary, i.e., abduction or kidnapping.

(4)   Juvenile - A person of any age who is missing and declared unemancipated as defined by the laws of his/her state of residence and does not meet the entry criteria set forth in 1, 2, 3, or 5.

(5)   Catastrophe : Victim - A person of any age who is missing after a disaster (U.S, Department of Justice, 1991).

The extensive Data Collection Entry Packet may be entered only by the originating agency which filed the initial report into the NCIC computer. Most law enforcement agencies are familiar with the procedure for entering a person into the NCIC system. However, some small town or rural law enforcement departments do not have a computer on site for submitting the information, nor the experience to do it. This limitation can be very frustrating for families. Their stress worsens if the agency is unwilling to ask for professional assistance and unfortunately this can, and does, happen.

If the originating agency is reluctant to get the Data Collection Entry Guide for a Missing Person, the family member can request the FBI to obtain the packet. Family members must follow the instructions carefully and fill out the appropriate answers. In turn, the missing person's doctor and dentist should fill out the medical questions, return the information to the originating agency, and request that they enter the information into the NCIC computer.

By law, when an adult disappears, the FBI does not become involved unless there is evidence of foul play across a state line. In contrast, when a child disappears, the FBI immediately becomes involved in the investigation. Missing adults, even those who are cognitively impaired, do not benefit from the same vigorous search resources as do children.

According to a **USA Today** report (Nameless Bodies

Burden, Baffle Law Enforcers," April 24, 1991) there may be as many as one thousand five hundred unidentified bodies nationwide who remain unidentified. The coroners who tag them as Jane or John Doe do not know where they came from, and families in search of missing persons do not know of their existence in a morgue. There is no requirement that all law enforcement agencies participate in informing NCIC when a body is found.

Family members are often desperately seeking to find a person, believing them to be alive, when, in fact, they may have been found injured or dead, but remain unidentified. When all search endeavors have proven fruitless and zero leads have surfaced, families should check with medical examiners. This is a dispirited undertaking, but a necessary one.

County medical examiners in all states are listed in **The National Directory of Addresses & Telephone Numbers**. Families may write to selected County Medical Examiners, inquiring if any unidentified bodies have been found and recorded in their jurisdiction.

The inquiry letter in Appendix 4 was mailed to numerous county medical examiners. Included with the letter was a self-addressed return postcard noting the specific agency contacted and whether the response was negative or positive for an unidentified body matching Stella Dickerman's description.

Journey Without End

For several months now, I have been blocked while trying to write the final thoughts for **Gone Without A Trace**. Suddenly, I realized there is no ending! As long as my mother remains unfound, as long as weary parents anguish for sons and daughters savagely taken, as long as thousands of older adults mysteriously disappear leaving families in despair, sifting for a single clue, the final words will be known only when the phone call comes with answers as to **what really happened.**

For Stella Dickerman, a missing person may represent someone in your life that you call 'mother', or someone that you call 'special friend'. In reading **Gone Without A Trace**, that terrible reality of someone suddenly disappearing becomes a little more vivid. For many people, this realization is unbearable to even ponder. It is a myth to believe it only happens to 'someone' else!

While writing **Gone Without A Trace**, a friend cautioned "Your feelings are personal... they belong to you, not into book form." It did not take long to realize how painful the reading of my story might be for some.

I believe strongly that real healing occurs only if a person is willing to face their grief and past losses. The burden of dealing with any loss becomes heavier when feelings are suppressed and not spoken about. It is my hope that anyone reading this book will be moved with the courage needed to heal from their accumulated losses in life. Most of all, I hope people will begin to talk to one another, in ways which are open, sincere and honest, and with the sensitivity and empathy necessary when speaking about personal pain.

With more and more families having to deal with a member suffering as a result of the wasting personhood associated with Alzheimer's and other memory impairments, it is crucial that the public understand how this disease manifests, and about its impact on families, friends and caregivers. All victims of Alzheimer's Disease and related disorders who become missing deserve the same conscientious efforts toward bringing them safely home, as do people unaffected by loss of memory. A missing person case cannot be closed, as long as the person remains unfound.

When the second Christmas season passed and my mother remained missing, a caring friend wrote: "I'm so sorry you had this difficult experience. It has been a real challenge to see any opportunity in this." Oftentimes, I have thought of these words... pondering what could be the challenge from my experience. I realize now that my mother's disappearance has propelled me to reach out to others faced with the tragedy of a family member *gone without a trace*. It is my hope that they will benefit from the telling of my experience.

I suggest to anyone suffering as a result of loss, take the risk of talking about your feelings to one another. This may give one unsuspecting soul permission to speak of painful feelings, which have been almost impossible to bear alone. The burden of loss may become a little lighter, if just one person feels less alone. This is what I envision for anyone reading ***Gone Without A Trace.***

AFTERWORD

Dear Reader:

At the time of press, on the third anniversary of my mother's disappearance, a hunter found her partial remains. Putting my struggles down in this book was one way to cope with my loss, finding her remains will help me move forward. I hope this story will be not only one of caution, but one of positive wisdom and tribute to a most extraordinary woman.

The author, Marianne Dickerman Caldwell may be
contacted at the address below.

Marianne Dickerman Caldwell
P.O. Box 1625
Pacifica,
CA. 94044-6625

Appendix 1

QUERY LETTER

October 16th, 1991

Dear Social Service Worker:

We are searching for an elderly woman, Stella Mallory Dickerman, our mother, who disappeared from Country School on Friday, September 13th, 1991. Despite three weeks of exhaustive searches of nearby forests, extensive newspaper and television coverage and the pursuit of several leads, we still have no idea of her whereabouts.

One possibility is that she was given a ride from the Rindge, New Hampshire area, and that she has been placed in a shelter, county or state hospital, or nursing home. She was carrying no identification, and because she suffers from Alzheimer's disease, may not have been able to give her name, address, or other identifying information. Although police have listed her name in the National Missing Persons Computer File, it is possible that she entered a shelter or hospital before the alert was issued. Or there may be another reason her identity has not been discovered.

Please check your records in case she passed through your program sometime after September 13th, 1991. If you have any leads, please call (Name of Originating Police Agency), at (list phone#), or one of us. Thank you very much for your help.

Sincerely,

Marianne Dickerman Caldwell   Name of Second
                                  Family Member

Address: Address:
Phone: Phone:

APPENDIX 2

MISSING PERSON PROFILE

Name: Stella Mallory Dickerman

Physical Description:
83 years old (appeared to most people to be in her 70's or even 60's)

Height 5'3"-5'5"   Weight 112 lbs.

Noticeably rounded shoulders from osteoporosis

Gray Hair (permanent Aug. '91)

Brown/Green eyes (hazel)

Right-handed

Excellent teeth, small chip off front tooth

Black mole in middle of back. Round black scar middle of left lower leg, recent cut middle of right lower leg.

Mild Rheumatoid arthritis affecting especially her back, hands and right wrist.

Wearing navy blue skirt, white blouse, white sweater, powder blue wind-breaker jacket, tan shoes with laces.

Was carrying a distinctive walking-stick (cane) with Alpine decorations (metal markings).

Behavior and Mannerisms:
Suffers from Alzheimer Disease.

Gentle, trusting, friendly. Readily asks for help. Appreciative of help.

Likes to talk, but confuses words. Forgets what she is saying. Disjointed conversations. Constantly changes topics. Might not be able to give full name or address. Significantly confused about time.

Easily becomes lost.

Packs and repacks suitcases or anything else. Frequently changes clothes.

Likes to walk and can walk long distance.

Conversation Topics:
Her family: (Son William, daughter Marianne, son Bob or Robert).

Her parents: (Her father who died suddenly of the flu, her mother who operated a college dormitory called 'The Vatican' in Oberlin, Ohio her former home) or Oberlin College.

Country school.

Water-color painting (she was an artist.)

Battle Creek, Michigan or Chautauqua Lake, New York.

Please Notify: Local police...name...phone number... List names of two family members and phone numbers.

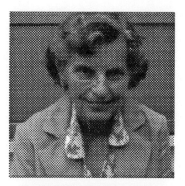

MISSING

Since 9/13/91
Stella Mallory Dickerman, an 83 year old woman with
Alzheimer's disorder, 5'4", 112 lbs., gray hair, hazel eyes

ALERT
If you find any of the following items, or have any information please contact the Rindge Police: (603) 899-5009

Wooden walking cane with metal
Austrian shields & "OZT"
 engraved on top.
Woman's light "sky blue"
 windbreaker jacket
tan shoes & navy blue skirt
white sweater & white blouse

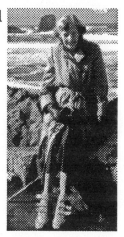

APPENDIX 4

LETTER TO MEDICAL EXAMINER

The following letter was mailed to numerous county medical examiners about Stella Dickerman. Included with the letter of inquiry was a self-addressed return postcard noting the specific agency contacted and whether the information available was negative or positive for an unidentified body meeting the description of Stella Dickerman.

TO: (Name) Office of County Medical Examiner

               Address

FROM: Name
               Address
               Phone

Re: **Unidentified Body**

I am writing with regard to my mother, Stella Mallory Dickerman, an eighty-three year old Alzheimer's disease victim who vanished September 13, 1991.

She walked away from a childrens' softball game at a boarding school located outside of Rindge, New Hampshire. The school is situated approximately one mile from the New Hampshire-Massachusetts border.

Despite an extensive search, immediately launched, of the area surrounding the school, no clues surfaced and she remains unfound. There is a possibility that she was given a ride out of the area, let out, died elsewhere or met foul play, and remains unidentified in a county morgue.

I have enclosed a self-addressed postcard for you to note your findings. I may be reached at the phone number listed for additional information.

Yours sincerely,

Marianne Caldwell

APPENDIX 5

IMPORTANT ORGANIZATIONS

Alzheimer's Disease and Related Disorders Association
919 N Michigan Avenue, Suite 1000,
Chicago, Illinois 60611-1676
PH: (800) 621-0379 (800) 272-3900
This organization provides literature on Alzheimer's
disease as well as referrals to local chapters.

Alzheimer Safe Return
C/O N.C.M.E.C. Attn: Hotline
2101 Wilson Rd. Suite 550
Arlington, VA 22201
PH: (800) 572-1122

National Institute on Aging
NIA Information Center
2209 Distribution Circle
Silver Springs, Maryland 20910
PH: (301) 496-1752

National Support Center For Families Of The Aging
P.O Box 245
Swarthmore
PA. 19081
PH: (215) 544-3605
This non-profit organization helps families cope with
their responsibilities to older relatives.

Family and Friends Of Missing Persons and Violent
Crime Victims
PO Box 21444
Seattle, Washington 98111

Kevin Collins Foundation
PO Box 590473
San Francisco, CA 94159
PH: (415) 771-8477

Polly Klaas Foundation
PO Box 800
Petaluma, CA 94953
PH: (800) 587-4357 or 1-707 769-1334
FAX: (707) 766-3824

National Center for Missing And Exploited Children
1835 K. Street NW, suite 700
Washington, D.C. 20006
PH: (800) 843-5678 or (206) 634-9821

National Child Identification Center, INC.
P.O.Box 3068A
Albuquerque,
New Mexico 87190
PH: (800) 222-4453

National Missing Children Hot Line
PH: (800) 843-5678 or (800) 621-4000

Search-A Central Registry Of The Missing
560 Sylvan Avenue
Englewood Cliffs,
N.J. 07632
This service provides information on missing individuals to law enforcement, security, medical and social service agencies.

APPENDIX 6

ALZHEIMER'S SAFE RETURN

The following is a list of Area Resource Centers for the Alzheimer's Association Safe Return Program:

St. Louis
Phone (314) 432-3422   Fax (314) 432-3824

Serving the states of—
  Illinois
  Iowa
  Kansas
  Michigan
  Minnesota
  Missouri
  Nebraska
  Oklahoma
  Texas
  Wisconsin

Louisville
Phone (502) 893-3607   Fax (502) 893-9635

Serving the states of——
    Delaware
    District of Columbia
    Indiana
    Kentucky
    Maryland
    Ohio
    Tennessee
    Virginia
    West Virginia

Palm Beach
Phone (407) 392-1363   Fax (407) 368-9082

Serving the states of——
    Alabama
    Arkansas
    Florida
    Georgia
    Louisiana
    Mississippi
    North Carolina
    South Carolina

Los Angeles
Phone (213) 938-3370   Fax (213) 938-1036

Serving the states of——
Arizona
California
Colorado
Hawaii
Nevada
New Mexico
Utah

Columbia/Willamette
Phone (503) 229-7115 Fax (503) 725-1754

Serving the states of——
Alaska
Idaho
Montana
North Dakota
Oregon
South Dakota
Washington
Wyoming

New York City
Phone 212) 983-0700   Fax (212) 697-6158

Serving the states of——
>Connecticut
>Maine
>Massachusetts
>New Hampshire
>New Jersey
>New York
>Pennsylvania
>Rhode Island
>Vermont

APPENDIX 7

STATE AGENCIES ON AGING

ALABAMA

COMMISSION ON AGING
770 Washington Ave.
Montgomery   AL 36130   (205) 242-5743

ALASKA

OLDER ALASKANS COMMISSION
PO Box C, MS 0209
Juneau   AK 99811   (907) 465-3250

AMERICAN SAMOA

TERRITORIAL ADMINISTRATION ON AGING
Government of American Samoa
Page Pago   96799   (684) 633-1251

ARIZONA

AGING & ADULT ADMINISTRATION
Department of Economic Security
1400 W. Washington St.
Phoenix   AZ 85007   (602) 542-4446

ARKANSAS

DIVISION OF AGING & ADULT SERVICES
Suite 1417, Donaghey Plz S
7th & Main Sts
PO Box 1417/Slot 1412
Little Rock   AR 72203-1437   (501) 682-2441

CALIFORNIA

DEPARTMENT OF AGING
1600 K St
Sacramento CA 95814   (916) 322-3887

COLORADO

AGING & ADULT SERVICES
Department of Social Services
10th Floor, 1575 Sherman St
Denver   CO 80203-1714   (303) 866-3851

CONNECTICUT

DEPARTMENT ON AGING
175 Main St
Hartford   CT 06106   (203) 566-7772

DELEWARE

DIVISION OF AGING
Department of Health & Social Services
1901 N DuPont Hwy
New Castle   DE 19720   (302) 421-6791

DISTRICT OF COLUMBIA

OFFICE ON AGING
2nd Floor, 1424 K St NW
Washington DC 20005   (202) 724-5626

FLORIDA

OFFICE OF AGING & ADULT SERVICES
1317 Winewood Blvd
Tallahassee   FL 32301   (904) 488-8922

GEORGIA

OFFICE OF AGING
Department of Human Resources
Suite 632, 878 Peachtree St. NE
Atlanta GA 30309   (404) 894-5333

GUAM

DIVISION OF SENIOR CITIZENS
Department of Public Health & Social Services
PO Box 2816
Agana   96910   (671) 734-4361

HAWAII

EXECUTIVE OFFICE ON AGING
Suite 241, 335 Merchant St
Honolulu HI 96813   (808) 586-0100

IDAHO

OFFICE ON AGING
Suite 108, Statehouse
Boise   ID 83720   (208) 334-3833

ILLINOIS

DEPARTMENT ON AGING
421 E. Capitol Ave
Springfield   IL 62701   (217) 785-2870

INDIANA

DEPARTMENT OF HUMAN SERVICES
251 N Illinois St
PO Box 7083
Indianapolis   IN 46207-7083   (317) 232-7020

IOWA

DEPARTMENT OF ELDER AFFAIRS
Suite 236, Jewett Bldg
914 Grand Ave
Des Moines   IA 50319   (515) 281-5187

KANSAS

DEPARTMENT ON AGING
122-S, Docking State Office Bldg
915 SW Harrison
Topeka   KS 66612-1500   (913) 296-4986

KENTUCKY

DIVISION FOR AGING SERVICES
Department for Social Services
275 E Main St
Frankfort KY 40621   (502) 564-6930

LOUISIANA

GOVERNOR'S OFFICE OF ELDERLY AFFAIRS
PO Box 80374
Baton Rouge LA 70898-0374   (504) 925-1700

MAINE

BUREAU OF ELDER & ADULT SERVICES
State House, Sta 11
Augusta ME 04333   (207) 624-5335

MARYLAND

STATE AGENCY ON AGING
Suite 1004, 301 W. Preston St
Baltimore MD 21201   (301) 225-1102

MASSACHUSETTS

EXECUTIVE OFFICE OF ELDER AFFAIRS
38 Chauncy St
Boston   MA 02111   (617) 727-7750

MICHIGAN

OFFICES OF SERVICES TO THE AGING
PO Box 30026
Lansing   MI 48909   (517) 373-8230

MINNESOTA

MINNESOTA BOARD ON AGING
4th Floor, Human Services Bldg
444 Lafayette Rd
St Paul   MN 55155-3843   (612) 296-2770

MISSISSIPPI

COUNCIL ON AGING
421 W Pascagoula St
Jackson MS 39203-3524   (601) 949-2070

MISSOURI

DIVISION OF AGING
Department of Social Services
615 Howerton CT
PO Box 1337
Jefferson MO 65102-1337   (314) 751-3082

MONTANA

THE GOVERNOR'S OFFICE ON AGING
Suite 219, State Capital Bldg.
Helena MT 59620   (406) 444-3111

NEBRASKA

DEPARTMENT OF AGING
State Office Bldg
301 Centennial Mall S
Lincoln NE 68509   (402) 471-2306

NEVADA

DIVISION FOR AGING SERVICES
Department of Human Resources
Suite 114, 340 N 11th St
Las Vegas   NV 89101   (702) 687-4210

NEW HAMPSHIRE

DIVSION OF ELDERLY & ADULT SERVICES
Department of Health & Human Services
6 Hazen Dr
Concord   NH 03301   (603) 271-4394

NEW JERSEY

DIVISION ON AGING
Department of Community Affairs
S Broad & Front Sts
CN 807
Trenton   NJ 08625-0807   (609) 292-4833

NEW MEXICO

AGENCY ON AGING
4th Floor, La Villa Rivera Bldg
224 E Palace Ave
Santa Fe   NM 87501   (505) 827-7640

NEW YORK

STATE OFFICE FOR THE AGING
2 Empire State Plaza
Albany NY 12223-0001   (518) 474-4425

NORTH CAROLINA

DIVISION OF AGING
Department of Human Resources
693 Palmer Dr
Raleigh   NC 27626-0531   (919) 733-3983

NORTH DAKOTA

AGING SERVICES DIVISION
Department of Human Services
State Capitol Bldg
Bismarck   ND 58505   (701) 224-2577

OHIO

DEPARTMENT OF AGING
8th Floor, 50 W Broad St
Columbus OH 43266-0501   (614) 466-5500

OKLAHOMA

AGING SERVICES DIVISION
Department of Human Services
PO Box 25352
 Oklahoma City   OK 73125   (405) 521-2281

OREGON

SENIOR SERVICES DIVISION
313 Public Services Bldg
Salem   OR 97310   (503) 313-4728

PENNSYLVANIA

DEPARTMENT OF AGING
231 State St.
Harrisburg PA 17101   (717) 783-1550

PUERTO RICO

GERICULTURE COMMISSION
GOVERNORS OFFICE OF ELDERLY AFFAIRS
Box 11398
Santurce   PR 00910   (809) 722-2429

RHODE ISLAND

DEPARTMENT OF ELDERLY AFFAIRS
60 Pine St.
Providence RI 02903   (401) 277-2858

SOUTH CAROLINA
COMMISSION ON AGING
Suite B-500, 400 Arbor Lake Dr
Columbia SC 29223   (803) 735-0210

SOUTH DAKOTA

ADULT SERVICES & AGING
Richard F Kneip Bldg
700 Governors Dr
Pierre SD 57501-2291   (605) 773-3656

TENNESSEE

COMMISSION ON AGING
Suite 201, 706 Church St
Nashville   TN 37219-5573   (615) 741-2056

TEXAS

DEPARTMENT ON AGING
PO Box 12786, Capitol Sta
Austin   TX 78741-3702   (512) 444-2727

UTAH

DIVISION OF AGING & ADULT SERVICES
120 N. 200 W.
PO Box 45500
Salt Lake City   UT 84145-0500   (801) 538-3910

VERMONT

OFFICE ON AGING
103 S. Main St
Waterbury   VT 05676   (802) 241-2400

VIRGINIA

DEPARTMENT FOR THE AGING
10th Floor, 700 Center
700 E Franklin St
Richmond   VA 23219-2327   (804) 225-2272

VIRGIN ISLANDS

DEPARTMENT OF HUMAN SERVICES
19 Estate Diamond Frederick Sted
St Croix   VI 00840   (809) 772-4850

WASHINGTON

AGING & ADULT SERVICES ADMINISTRATION
Department of Social & Health Services
Main Stop 0B-44-A
Olympia WA 98504   (206) 586-3768

WEST VIRGINIA

COMMISSION ON AGING
State Capitol Complex
Holly Grove
Charleston WV 25305   (304) 348-3317

WISCONSIN

BUREAU ON AGING
DEPARTMENT OF HEALTH & SOCIAL SERVICES
PO BOX 7851
Madison   WI 53707   (608) 266-2536

WYOMING

COMMISSION ON AGING
1st Floor, Hathaway Bldg
Cheyenne   WY 82002   (307) 777-7986

Source: U.S. DHSS/HCFA

Appendix 8

Monadnock Ledger,

Peterborough, NH, 9-19-91

Rindge Woman Is Still Missing
Officials Call Off Intensive Search for 83-Year Old Alzheimer's Sufferer

Rindge—After five days, officials have called off the search for 83-year old Stella Dickerman, an Alzheimer's Disease sufferer who walked away from a softball game at the Hampshire Country School on Friday afternoon and hasn't been seen since.

The intense search involved tracking dogs, teams from several different local, state and federal agencies, and many volunteers.

"I don't think any of us have been getting much sleep, Rindge firefighters Auxiliary member Delores Schneider said Monday afternoon. "The sound of the rain on the roof wakes you and you think of the possibility that the poor woman might be out there. You can't get back to sleep with that thought in your head."

Now that the search is ending, state and local police have taken over and are investigating any and all leads. Anyone who thinks they might have seen Stella Dickerman or has any information is urged to contact the Rindge police at 899-5009.

Dickerman was a new Rindge resident. She moved here two weeks ago from Oberlin, Ohio, and had been living with her son William, a director and teacher at the Hampshire

Country School.

Dickerman is 5 foot six and about 115 pounds. When she walked away at 4.30p.m. Friday, she was wearing a navy blue skirt, a light blue nylon jacket over a white sweater and light brown shoes. She was carrying a distinctive Alpine walking stick decorated with metal tokens.

When it was discovered that she was missing, school officials and students conducted a search. When she couldn't be located, authorities were notified.

At 8.30p.m. the New Hampshire Fish and Game Department took over the search. State police tracking dogs, bloodhounds and German Shepherds were brought in and worked through the night and into Saturday. They were unable to locate the woman.

Temperatures Friday night dropped to 45 degrees and it rained. During the day Saturday, almost 100 searchers—members of the fish and game department, various local fire and police departments, as well as volunteers—went over the area, clambering for hours through the wet brush and swamps.

A National Guard helicopter flew over fields, Beaver Pond and two nearby lakes. Late Saturday afternoon, six new dogs, from the New England K-9 Search and Rescue Unit and trained to pick up scents by sniffing the air, started work and continued through late Sunday morning, but to no avail.

Then between 50 and 60 searchers—many of whom had participated in the cold, wet exhausting effort Saturday, too—tried again. At about 5p.m., the day's last search was done and still there was nothing.

On Tuesday, New England K-9 Search and Rescue continued the search, deploying three dogs throughout the day.

KEENE SENTINEL

Keene, NH, 9-20-94

SKULL FOUND; MYSTERY ENDS

Body part is that of woman missing 3 years from Rindge

New Ipswich—A skull found Saturday in New Ipswich woods was that of an 83-year old woman who wandered away from a Rindge boarding school three years ago.

Dental records prove that the skull is Stella Dickerman's, said Lt. Gerard Bernier of the N.H. Fish and Game Department.

Dickerman was in the mid stages of Alzheimer's when she disappeared, said her son, William Dickerman, admission director at Hampshire Country School in Rindge.

A Massachusetts bow hunter found the skull Saturday on Barrett Mountain in New Ipswich, a little more than a mile from the school campus in eastern Rindge, Bernier said.

"For me, it's the resolution I would have hoped for," William Dickerman said. "It's nice to have the finality. But it's also nice to know she died in the woods instead of having been abducted or given a ride and ended up in the homeless section of Boston."

He said he suspects his mother was cold, scared and lonely when she died, but he preferred that to a violent abduction.

"It's hard to think what they found or how they found her," said Dickerman's daughter, Marianne Caldwell, who lives in California.

Stella Dickerman wandered away in the late afternoon of September 13, 1991, setting off a massive search that involved dogs, helicopters, divers and hundreds of volunteers.

101

During the past three years, Stella Dickerman's family and friends had searched the woods near the campus periodically, and had also distributed flyers and enlisted news-media assistance, trying to jog the memory of anyone who might have seen Dickerman on that day or given her a ride.

Just a few weeks ago, Caldwell wrote a letter to the Sentinel, reminding people of the continued search for information about her mother's disappearance.

Monday's discovery brings some relief. "I'm not wondering now—I know that it's over and it certainly is not what I had ever thought about," Caldwell said this morning from California. "But, it certainly has brought some answers, not all of them, but it's helped a great deal."

Though her mother had been missing for more than three years, and the family had taken steps to have her declared legally dead, Caldwell said there was still a slight glimmer that Stella Dickerman might be found alive.

"Probably 98% of me knew that she wasn't alive, but without any information one always does wonder," said Caldwell, who's written a book about her mother's disappearance. "That was the part that was so troubling. But I know it's over for her, she's not in distress and now I'll be able to go on."

Family members feared she may have been abducted, and they cringed every time they heard a news report about an abduction, William Dickerman said.

The skull was found in a grove of maple trees on Barret Mountain. No other bones or clothing were found. Dickerman said his mother liked the woods, and had explored the Barrett Mountain area with him for years.

Suggested Reading

Aronson, M. (1988) **Understanding Alzheimer's Disease.** New York: Charles Scribner's Sons

Figley, C.R. (1985) **Trauma and It's Wake.** New York: Bruner/Mazel

Forsythe, E. (1990) **Alzheimer's Disease: The Long Bereavement.** Winchester: Faber & Faber Inc.,

Kushner, H. (1981) **When Bad Things Happen to Good People.** New York: Schocken Books

Mace, N., & Rabins, P. (1991) **The 36-Hour Day: A Family Guide to Caring for Persons with Alzheimer's Disease, Related Dementing Illnesses, and Memory Loss in Later Life.** Baltimore: The John Hopkins University Press

Powell, L., & Courtice, K. (1992 Rev. Ed.) **Alzheimer's Disease: A Guide for Families.** Palo Alto: Addison-Wesley Publishing Co. Inc.

Raphael, B. (1984) **The Anatomy of Bereavement.** New York: Basic Books

Stearns, A. (1984) **Living Through Personal Crisis.** Chicago: The Thomas More Press

Tatelbaum, J. **The Courage to Grieve: Creative Living, Recovery, and Growth through Grief.** New York: Harper Collins

References

Bowlby, J. (1980) **Attachment and Loss.** (Vol. III: Loss) New York: Basic Books.

Frankl, V. (1963) **Man's Search for Meaning.** New York: Washington Square Press.

Gill, K. (1993) **The National Directory of Addresses and Telephone Numbers.** Detroit: Omnigraphics, Inc.

Gunderson, T. (1989) **How to Locate Anyone Anywhere.** New York: E.P. Dutton

Herman, J. (1992) **Trauma and Recovery.** Basic Books Division of HarperCollins.

Lukas, C. and Seiden, H. (1987) **Silent Grief.** New York: Charles Scribner's Sons.

U.S. Department of Justice **Missing Person File-Data Collection Entry Guide For Families.** Federal Bureau of Investigation: National Crime Information Center.

Verrier, N (1993) **The Primal Wound**. Baltimore: Gateway Press, Inc.

Viorst, J. (1986) **Necessary Losses**. New York: Ballantine Books.

Other Titles from Elder Books

Failure-Free Activities for the Alzheimer's Patient
by Carmel Sheridan

This award-winning book shows you how to raise the quality of life for patients and caregivers through simple meaningful activities. The author describes how to focus on the abilities that remain rather than the person's deficits. Hundred of activities are outlined which help to raise self-esteem and relieve boredom and frustration. Now in its thirteenth U.S. printing, *Failure-Free Activities* is recognised internationally as a groundbreaking activity book and has been translated into Spanish, Dutch and Japanese.
$10.95

Reminiscence: Uncovering A lifetime of Memories
by Carmel Sheridan

Written in easily-understood language, this book shows how to use reminiscence with the well and confused elderly in the home, in day care, social centers and hospitals. 164 pages packed with activities and ways to uncover memories.
$11.95

Surviving Alzheimer's
by Florian Raymond

Written by a family caregiver, this is an essential book for those closest to the Alzheimer's patient. Reader friendly, **Surviving Alzheimer's** describes in simple terms how caregivers can renew and restore themselves during the up and downs of caregiving. A treasure house of practical tips, ideas and survival strategies, the book shows caregivers how to take care of themselves as well as the patient. It outlines dozens of coping skills and ways to help maintain health throughout the difficult caregiving journey.
$10.95

Activity Ideas for the Budget Minded
by Debra Cassistre

Already used by thousands of activity directors, this new edition is packed with dozens of hands-on, ready to use budget-stretching activities. These low-cost activity ideas will give your program an inexpensive boost, create variety and give residents the kind of stimulation they deserve
$10.95

Tell Me A Story
Tell Me A Story is a remarkably simple kit for family caregivers who find it difficult to initiate conversation with an Alzheimer's patient. A set of 56 cue cards, the kit is designed specially to encourage communication through reminiscence, storytelling and some role play. An ideal companion to Carmel Sheridan's book **Reminiscence**.
$10.95

Gone Without A Trace

by Marianne Dickerman Caldwell

On Friday, September 13, 1991, Stella Mallory Dickerman, an Alzheimer's victim, wandered away from a school softball match and was never seen again.

"To learn how to prevent such a disappearance, or what to do if it occurs, be sure to read **Gone Without A Trace.**"

Joe Klaas, **The Twelve Steps To Happiness.**

"Touching insights into the experience of losing a loved one to Alzheimer's disease and then, losing her again, without knowing whether she ever will be found. **Gone Without A Trace** is an exceptional true story."

Suzanne Hanser, Ed. D. Alzheimer's Association, Palo Alto, CA

The first book published to chronicle the experience of loss and bereavement when a loved one vanishes and remains missing. Providing step-by-step guidelines, the author shows how to mobilize a search for a missing adult.
$10.95

Caregivers Catalog

An essential catalog of resources especially for caregivers of the elderly. Books, tapes, videos and activity resources to raise the quality of life for caregiver and patient.
FREE

ORDER FORM

Mail To:
Elder Books
PO Box 490, Forest Knolls, CA 94933

QUANTITY	TITLE	PRICE
_____	**Surviving Alzheimer's**	$10.95
_____	**Failure-Free Activities for the Alzheimer's Patient**	$10.95
_____	**Reminiscence**	$10.95
_____	**Activity Ideas for the Budget Minded**	$10.95
_____	**Tell Me A Story**	$10.95
_____	**Gone Without A Trace**	$10.95
_____	**Caregivers Catalog**	FREE

Name _____

Address _____

City _____

State _____ Zip _____

Telephone:_____

Shipping:$2.50 for first book. Additional books: $1.00 each
California residents please add 8.5% California Sales Tax.